W9-CCD-095

Dan B. Allender, Ph.D.

THE
HEALING
PATH

A STUDY GUIDE BASED ON THE BOOK

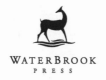

WaterBrook
PRESS

A Study Guide
to THE HEALING PATH by Dan Allender
PUBLISHED BY WATERBROOK PRESS
12265 Oracle Boulevard, Suite 200
Colorado Springs, Colorado 80921

Quotations from *The Healing Path:* © 1999 by Dr. Dan B. Allender

Scripture quotations, unless otherwise indicated, are taken from the *Holy Bible, New International Version®. NIV®.* Copyright © 1973, 1978, 1984 by International Bible Society. Used by permission of Zondervan Publishing House. All rights reserved. Also quoted, *The New Revised Standard Version Bible* (NRSV) © 1989 by the Division of Christian Education of the National Council of the Churches of Christ in the United States of America. Used by permission. All rights reserved.

ISBN 978-1-57856-156-8

Copyright © 1999 by WaterBrook Press

Published in association with the literary agency of Alive Communications, Inc. 7680 Goddard Street, Suite 200, Colorado Springs, CO 80920

All rights reserved. No part of this book may be reproduced or transmitted in any form or by any means, electronic or mechanical, including photocopying, recording, or by any information storage and retrieval system, without permission in writing from the publisher.

Published in the United States by WaterBrook Multnomah, an imprint of the Crown Publishing Group, a division of Random House Inc., New York.

WATERBROOK and its deer colophon are registered trademarks of Random House Inc.

Printed in the United States of America

THE LONG WALK

A companion study to Chapter 1
in THE HEALING PATH

In this opening session you will think about your most common responses to suffering. You'll also think about how people close to you deal with suffering. The spotlight in this study will be on you, so it will be important not to evade looking at yourself by focusing on others' faults. Still, when you consider how others help or harm you by their response to suffering, it may be easier for you to see how your stance toward suffering truly affects the people around you.

If you are meeting with a group and don't already know each other well, take some time to introduce yourselves at the beginning of the meeting. You will be sharing very personal things, so it will be important to lay a foundation of trust. You'll be telling your stories at some length in session 2, so you don't need to do that now. Instead, use question 1 as a chance to tell others one thing about your life that motivates you to study the healing path.

Of course we know suffering will visit us sometimes, but we don't want to think about it. What is the point of contemplating something that is out of our control? If we could prevent it, then we might briefly consider our stance toward suffering. But why bother when God "causes the sun to rise on the evil and the good, and sends rain on the righteous and the unrighteous" (Matthew 5:45)? We're all going to get our share of joy and sorrow, so let's just get on with our lives and hope for the best.

The problem with this position is that once the inevitable pain comes, it is too late to consider how we will allow ourselves to be shaped by it.

—Dan Allender in THE HEALING PATH

1. What motivates you to take a long look at how you respond to suffering? What do you hope to get out of this study?

The Healing Path is about how God redeems our doubt and betrayal, our despair and powerlessness, our disappointment and ambivalence. It calls us to move toward the great destination of this life: becoming a man or woman of faith, hope, and love.

—Dan Allender in THE HEALING PATH

2. What is your immediate, gut reaction to the statement, "To live is to hurt"?

3. Dr. Allender lists four common responses to pain. In the following checklist, mark the statements that sound like you.

PARANOID: "LIFE IS DIFFICULT, THEN YOU DIE."

- ☐ I see the dark lining in every cotton-candy cloud.
- ☐ I'm often cynical.
- ☐ My preferred form of humor is irony—dark and somewhat bitter.
- ☐ I enjoy books and films with tragic endings.
- ☐ I compete to survive.
- ☐ I prefer to expect the worst rather than to be surprised by it.
- ☐ I'm terrified of hoping in something I can't control.
- ☐ I avoid taking the risk of pursuing my deepest dreams because the chance of success is so slim, and I fear disappointment and failure.

FATALISTIC: "QUÉ SERÁ, SERÁ—ROLL WITH IT, BABY."

- ☐ I just relax and let things come.
- ☐ I believe in "Let go and let God."
- ☐ I don't take criticism personally or seriously.
- ☐ I rarely seek constructive criticism.
- ☐ People find me pleasant, but unwilling to engage in conflict or difficult conversations.
- ☐ I avoid confronting those who harm me.
- ☐ I'm more interested in surviving life unscathed than in learning from it.
- ☐ Nothing much bothers me.
- ☐ I rarely worry.
- ☐ I rarely look back.
- ☐ I have few passionate desires for anything.
- ☐ I'm not very intimate with anyone.

- [ ] Feeling other people's pain is not my strength.
- [ ] I don't have a strong sense of calling and purpose for my life.
- [ ] Nothing I've suffered has been all that serious.

HEROIC: "WHAT DOES NOT KILL ME MAKES ME STRONGER."

- [ ] I view suffering as a challenge to be overcome.
- [ ] I like to feel I'm in charge of myself and my destiny.
- [ ] Some people find me controlling or domineering.
- [ ] Weak people annoy me.
- [ ] I am a conqueror, not a victim.
- [ ] My motto is, "No whining."
- [ ] I often want to shout, "Just do it!"
- [ ] My family, friends, and/or coworkers have trouble keeping up with me.
- [ ] My spouse/girlfriend/boyfriend is lonely.
- [ ] I don't like the idea of needing someone else's sacrificial support.
- [ ] I like to rely on myself.

OPTIMISTIC: "JUST GRIN AND BEAR IT."

- [ ] I laugh at suffering.
- [ ] I expect good things to happen to me, and generally they do.
- [ ] When people suffer, I tell them to think positively.
- [ ] I'd rather help someone solve problems than just listen to him tell his tale of woe.
- [ ] I don't think about the poor much.
- [ ] I expect everything to work out for the best, so there's not much point in dwelling on the bad things.
- [ ] I don't know anyone with severe problems that cannot be solved in this life.
- [ ] I don't think about death much.

4. How would you summarize your most common response to suffering in your own life?

5. How would you summarize your most common response to someone else's suffering?

6. Think about the people in your most intimate relationships. How do they respond to suffering? Write their names next to the labels, "Paranoid," "Fatalistic," "Heroic," and "Optimistic" above.

7. How do these people's approaches to suffering affect your relationships with them?

The way we approach suffering usually is determined by our basic attitude toward the struggles of this life. Many of us believe that God's commitment is to help us avoid or triumph over adversity—we are "more than conquerors." And we are. But that biblical belief can be cheapened to presume there is a way to completely eradicate our pain if we just find the right combination of prayer and action.

—Dan Allender in THE HEALING PATH

Romans 1–8 is Paul's long discourse on what God is up to in sending Christ and the Holy Spirit into the world. In the second half of Romans 8, Paul brings this discourse to a climax. He writes in the context of his own expertise in suffering—he has been jailed, beaten, betrayed, and robbed; he has been hungry, sick, cold, and wet; he has numerous enemies and few possessions.

Read Romans 8:17-39.

8. List each statement Paul makes in this passage about suffering (including frustration, bondage, groaning, hardship, and so on).

9. What arguments does this passage offer *for* or *against* the belief that God promises to eradicate our pain if we pray and act rightly?

10. According to Paul, what good things can we attain through our suffering?

11. What do you think Paul means in verse 37 when he calls us "more than conquerors"? In the context of this passage, what does conquering involve?

12. What does Paul want us to *believe* in the midst of our suffering?

13. What does Paul want us to *do* in response to our suffering?

14. What help does God offer as we suffer?

15. What, in your view, is the point of contemplating suffering, since so often it is out of your control?

16. Write a prayer to God, expressing what you hope he will do in your heart as you study *The Healing Path*. Tell God some of the thoughts and feelings inside you as you begin this study.

THE HEALING PATH

*A companion study to Chapter 2
in* THE HEALING PATH

This session offers an overview of the desert experience. By reflecting on your own story in light of the story of Lamentations, you will begin to discern some of the landmarks of your desert—betrayal, powerlessness, and ambivalence—along with their corresponding spiritual struggles. If you are meeting with a group, you will have a chance to tell some of your story and hear the stories of others.

The healing path must pass through the desert or
else our healing will be the product of our own will
and wisdom. It is in the silence of the desert that we
hear our dependence on noise. It is in the poverty of
the desert that we see clearly our attachments to the
trinkets and baubles we cling to for security and
pleasure. The desert shatters the soul's arrogance and
leaves body and soul crying out in thirst and hunger.
In the desert, we trust God or we die.

—Dan Allender in THE HEALING PATH

---

1. All of us have encountered suffering in small or large ways. Have you ever told anyone about your suffering? If so, how have they responded?

2. When you think now about telling others about some hard part of your life, what thoughts and feelings come to mind?

BETRAYAL

Betrayal, whether the result of mutual failings or one party's error, leaves the heart sick over the past and fearful of future loss. When the past is littered with the rusted-out remains of broken friendships, the heart is robbed of the desire to trust—not only in the relationship that has suffered harm, but in all other relationships. Betrayal particularly throws into question our relationship with God. Does he rescue? Does he protect? Will he let the guilty go free?

—Dan Allender in THE HEALING PATH

---

3. In your own words, how would you define betrayal?

4. How does betrayal shake our faith in God?

5. Describe an experience you have had of betrayal.

6. How did that experience, and/or experiences like it, encourage you to doubt God's goodness, justice, or commitment to protect you?

POWERLESSNESS

Hope is by far one of the most dangerous commit-
ments we make in life. Hope draws us to create and
sacrifice without any guarantee of fulfillment. The
more we hope, the more we lean into the future,
risking the present to secure the dreams that entice
us. No wonder a wound like the loss of a job, or a
rape, sears us with the foolishness of anticipating the
future. "Once burned, shame on you. Twice burned,
shame on me." For many, the shame of hoping and
being burned again and again has turned them
against hope and solidified their commitment to find
something in this life they can control.

—Dan Allender in THE HEALING PATH

7. In your own words, how would you define hope?

8. How does suffering discourage us from hoping?

9. Describe a time when you felt powerless.

10. How did this experience of powerlessness, and/or others like it, encourage you to abandon hope?

AMBIVALENCE

Ambivalence is feeling torn in two. It creates a divided sense of self that feels shame and self-hatred for once enjoying what is ultimately stained or stolen from us....

Ambivalence exposes our heart's desire for what we are no longer free to enjoy. It causes us to question the sanity of giving and receiving pleasure in our work and relationships. What if it ends? What if

I enjoy you more than you enjoy me? What if your delight in me is bogus? Or worse, what if it is mere manipulation to get from me what you want? What if I love you and then you die, divorce me, or turn against me? The risk is more than I can bear, and so I refuse to open my heart to another person who will arouse my desire and then might use me or dash me to the ground.

—Dan Allender in THE HEALING PATH

11. Think about those situations in which you felt betrayed and powerless. Do you feel ashamed to have once enjoyed your betrayer, or the person or situation that left you powerless? Describe any mixed feelings you have about the people involved.

12. How does this kind of ambivalence discourage us from loving freely again?

13. Have those times of betrayal, powerlessness, and ambivalence hindered your ability to love deeply? If so, in what ways do you hold back from love?

14. In what ways did God feed and protect you in the midst of these painful circumstances? How did you experience his compassion or faithfulness, even if you didn't recognize him at the time?

Some of us find it embarrassing to tell these stories of humiliation and even more shameful to admit the ways they have sapped our faith, hope, and love. The writers of the Bible, however, were unashamed to tell such stories.

The book of Lamentations is an intricate poem written to express intense grief. The writer (probably the prophet Jeremiah) has witnessed the siege of Jerusalem in which the city's inhabitants have been slowly starved into surrendering to the Babylonian invaders. After many months, the Babylonians have finally taken Jerusalem and subjected its inhabitants to slaughter, rape, mutilation, and slavery. The poet details the wreckage, not flinching from describing cannibalism and children dying of famine in the streets.

The climax of the poem is chapter 3. Here the poet speaks not just of Jerusalem's suffering, but of his own. On top of everything else, his own people have betrayed him (Jeremiah was imprisoned for treason because he predicted that God would allow the city's defeat). Read Lamentations 3:1-33, preferably aloud.

15. Read the passage again, this time looking for what the poet says about each of the following experiences:

a. betrayal

b. doubt of God

c. faith in God

d. powerlessness

e. despair

f. hope

g. ambivalence toward God emotionally

16. The poem is full of ambivalence: love for those who are now dead, and pain over that love. Read Lamentations 2:11-13. Imagine yourself in a situation like that. What would it take for you to risk loving people again after losing so many loved ones to a violent and ugly death?

17. What do you find in the poet's convictions about God (Lamentations 3:22-33) that might have helped him risk loving again?

18. In questions 1 through 14 above, you thought about your own story. Perhaps it seems inconsequential compared to the destruction of Jerusalem, or perhaps you find it easy to identify with the poet of Lamentations. In what ways does the poet's story help you make sense of your story?

19. Think about your own affliction and wandering (3:19). As God listens to your story, what do you think he wants to say to you? Is there anything in Lamentations that sounds like God speaking to you?

This poet labored to make a work of art from his grief. In each chapter of the poem, successive verses begin with successive letters of the Hebrew alphabet. Clearly, this poet spent considerable time reflecting on—even wallowing in—his traumatic story. Later generations of Jews up to the present day have used Lamentations to help them do the same thing.

20. What do you think is the benefit of writing or telling one's "lamentations" as a story for others to hear? Why invest the effort?

If you are meeting with a group, your answers to questions 3-14 can form the basis of a story you can tell your group. Depending on the size of the group and the time you have, allow each person five to ten minutes to tell as much of his or her story as each wishes to tell. It will be most helpful if you talk about one or two incidents that represent your experience of betrayal, powerlessness, ambivalence, and their effects, rather than giving a general overview of your life. If the image of desert or valley helps you, use them to talk about silence, poverty, danger, or aloneness.

By the end of your study of *The Healing Path*, you will be telling the redemptive sides of your stories—the ways in which God has used your experiences to deepen faith, hope, and love in you. If you already can tell that part of your story, feel free to do so. You may want to talk about how God fed or protected you in your desert or valley. However, don't feel pressured to give your story a happy ending, and don't use redemption to gloss over the painful parts of your story. For now, it may be most helpful for the group to hear of your desert experience.

If you feel that you express yourself better through pictures or objects than through words, you might make a collage or bring some old photographs or childhood possessions with which to tell your story to the group.

21. As you end your study, take a few minutes to "sit alone in silence" (Lamentations 3:28) and contemplate both the truth of your desert and the truth of the Lord's faithfulness in it. Ask God to reveal his compassion to you.

EMBRACING LIFE

A companion study to Chapter 3
in THE HEALING PATH

Dr. Allender likens the healing path to an embrace. In this session you will look at the four elements of an embrace:

- Opening the heart rather than cynically shutting down.
- Waiting with anticipation rather than killing hope.
- Encircling others instead of standing alone.
- Letting go of the moment.

OPENING THE HEART

If we don't open our arms and hearts to the past, we will remain suspicious and closed in the present.... What does opening our arms to the past require? Embracing life in a fallen world, especially as we face the past, means honoring the data of life by actively turning toward the whole truth, reaching out to meet it, while also making space in our heart to receive it.

—Dan Allender in THE HEALING PATH

1. When you think about opening your arms to the truth about your past, what feelings and thoughts well up from inside you?

2. What do you think opening your arms to the past involves for you personally at this stage of your growth?

3. What (if anything) motivates you to open your arms to the pain of your past or present?

4. How has God opened his arms to you and your struggle?

WAITING WITH ANTICIPATION

Waiting stirs the soul's deep struggle with hope. We think it pleasant to hope, but in fact, nothing is more difficult than to hope. Hope lifts us up and gives us a view of how much ground must still be traveled on our journey. It allows us to see the horizon, usually far beyond our reach.

Oddly, hope both illumines what we most want to achieve and distances us from it. If we run to the horizon, it recedes. Many run anyway, striving to fully comprehend, seeking an alternative to living with uncertainty. Others refuse to dream at all, fleeing the potential disappointment of having their desires dashed.

—Dan Allender in THE HEALING PATH

5. At those times when waiting is difficult, which of these tempts you more: the refusal to live with uncertainty or the refusal to dream? How does that refusal typically show itself in your life?

6. Have you ever looked for quick fixes to your hungers? If so, what sorts of quick fixes have you tried?

7. Is God making you wait now? If so, how can you let this time of waiting draw you closer to God?

> We are meant to encircle another, not with a vice
> grip that asserts our power or preeminence, nor with
> a limp squeeze that refuses to really hold the other in
> our arms. Encircling another calls us to both receive
> and to give through an interplay of honor, passion,
> and respect. The interplay is full of mystery in its
> process and outcome.
>
> —Dan Allender in THE HEALING PATH

8. When was the last time you encircled another person with honor, passion, or respect? Describe the emotions you felt.

9. Have you ever sensed God encircling you in his embrace? If so, tell a little about that experience. If not, what's it like for you to read about it when it hasn't happened to you?

An embrace from God or from another is life giving
and heart changing. Once we receive it, we never
want to let go. We want people to stay and moments
to last. One of the hardest components of life is saying farewell and letting sweet moments fade. And the
more meaningful the experience, the harder it is to
open our arms and let the moment go. For that rea-
son it is easy to let go too soon. Often we brush
away the precious touch too quickly and refuse to let
our desire grow. Or we grip the moment with frantic
craving and end up crushing it in our arms.

—Dan Allender in THE HEALING PATH

10. Is it hard for you to let sweet moments with God
go, or to give people in your life space? What is it
about letting go that you sometimes find difficult?

The book of Deuteronomy is a set of sermons delivered
by Moses as the Israelites camped just outside the
Promised Land. The people stood on the brink of a decision that would consume the rest of their lives and their
children's lives. Would they venture into years of struggle
to occupy the land promised to them but not yet delivered? Or would they hang back? Near the end of the
book, Moses states the choice to follow God or not to

follow him as a stark choice between life and death. "Choose life," Moses urged the people, but the choice was theirs.

Read Deuteronomy 30:9-15,19-20.

11. How did Moses describe the "life" he was asking the people to choose?

12. What actions were involved in choosing life?

13. What promises did Moses make on God's behalf if the people chose life?

14. The Lord promised to make Israel prosper if the people obeyed his call to choose life. But that prosperity would take years to accomplish. Along the way there would be many battles with fierce Canaanites, as well as mundane but backbreaking labor, such as clearing land for farming and building homes. How is God's call to choose life similar for you?

15. Is "life" worth that much to you? Or is God's offer of life attractive only if it can come quickly and easily?

16. Tell God what you currently think about this call to choose life. Tell him your hopes and fears and what you feel when you face the prospect of waiting and struggling. If your arms are open to his embrace, tell him so; if not, tell him why you're not yet willing to open your arms.

17. What is one concrete gesture of embracing life that you can make this week? If you can't think of something right now, be alert this week for an opportunity.

BETRAYAL AND THE LOSS OF FAITH

*A companion study to Chapter 4
in THE HEALING PATH*

In this session you will examine betrayal, its harmful effects, and its opportunities for growth. You will find it helpful to focus on one specific experience of betrayal—either a single event or a series of encounters with a particular person or group. In this way, you will be able to practice an approach to reflecting on betrayal that you can apply to other experiences.

Sessions 4 through 6 will ask you to tell some difficult stories. If you meet with a group, you may want to check in with each other briefly before diving into this material. At the beginning of each of these sessions, for example, you could ask each person to tell briefly what it was like to work through that session's material. What thoughts and feelings came up? How did the material interact with the rest of your life?

Essentially, betrayal is the breaking of an implied or stated commitment of care. We are to love the Lord our God with our whole heart, soul, strength, and mind, and to love our neighbor as ourselves. We are to care—that is, internally orient our heart toward and act on behalf of others for their good. We are to

care for God. We are to care for others. When we
break covenant toward another and refuse to care,
then we have betrayed ourselves, our God, and that
person.

—Dan Allender in THE HEALING PATH

1. In the experience that comes to mind, how were
you betrayed?

2. How was your dignity effaced, marred, mocked,
manipulated, or ignored in that experience?

3. Did you respond by refusing to care or hope for
good for the person(s) who betrayed you? If so, how
did that refusal play itself out?

4. Do you think that looking at your own lack of love in this situation amounts to blaming the victim? Explain your view on this.

5. Dr. Allender says, "All betrayal is a community affair." How were other people drawn into the betrayal you experienced?

People who have been betrayed often experience nausea. It is as if they have lost their footing and suffer the roiling seasickness of a world that has lost its foundation. Not only does betrayal rip away the foundation of trust and confidence in others, but it also isolates us in a web of memories....

Why is memory so closely connected to betrayal? Memory is our map for living life. We may know the terrain from home to work so well that we don't even seem to need to turn the wheel of the car; it happens without thought or apparent choice. But what happens when a detour takes us out of familiar territory to a part of town that is both new and scary? We take out a map to find our way.

—Dan Allender in THE HEALING PATH

---

6. How have you been tormented by memories—either good or bad ones—because of this betrayal?

7. How do memories of this experience affect you now?

8. Have you done anything—such as cutting ties to the past or avoiding discussing those times—in order to protect yourself from painful memories? If so, what have you done?

Doubt is an acid that eats away at our stories. As the questions about what happened and what we did wrong multiply, our stories dissolve and we lose the confidence that those stories once provided. Doubt paralyzes us and makes even the simple decisions of life seem herculean....

Doubt is a form of doublethink that paralyzes us with the myriad options, the potential harm of another bad choice, and the shame that waits if we are mistaken again.

—Dan Allender in THE HEALING PATH

---

9. In what ways do you struggle with doubting yourself or God?

10. Do you find it hard to make decisions? If so, what kinds of decisions are hardest for you?

11. Do you ever feel numb? If you do, talk about the last time you were aware of numbness.

Our heart aches for good things, legitimate desires. And when God refuses to act to keep those desires alive, we find that our faith falters. Sometimes it dies. When faith withers, so does our capacity to remember his redemption with awe and gratitude.

The result of lost faith is a refusal to remember, and therefore a loss of confidence and energy to tackle the daily ups and downs of life.... A loss of faith often leads to a distant, rule-bound relationship with God that does not stray but also does not desire. Life without faith becomes anemic and pre-dictable, never sufficiently stirring to compel us to risk for the future.

—Dan Allender in THE HEALING PATH

---

12. Would you describe your relationship with God as distant, rule-bound, or lacking in strong desire? What are the signs in your life that this is or isn't true for you?

The Psalms are songs written by poets who struggle. The psalmists express the range of human emotions, and sometimes their honest anger and even vengefulness shock us. There is nothing distant or rule-bound in the relationship between God and the poet of Psalm 55, for example. His desires are strong, and with great frankness he pours out both his anguish at betrayal and his determination to find his way back to faith.

Read Psalm 55.

13. How does the writer of Psalm 55 describe his experience of betrayal?

14. How does he describe his emotional responses to this betrayal?

15. What do you make of his wish, expressed in verse 15: "Let death take my enemies by surprise;/let them go down alive to the grave,/for evil finds lodging among them"? For instance, does this seem like an unchristian sentiment? Can you identify with it?

16. Do you think God prefers to deal with someone who rages like this psalmist or with someone who is dutiful but numb? Why?

17. How does the psalmist express his faith in the midst of his many strong emotions?

18. Read aloud a verse or several verses from this psalm that express what you feel or desire regarding your betrayal and/or your current relationship with God. Don't choose the verses that express where you think you *should* be or how you think you *should* feel. Choose those that express where you actually are right now regarding doubt or faith, fear or courage, anger or peace.

The fruit of facing betrayal in others and ourselves is that we come to a new awareness of God's faithfulness in response to our betrayal of him. He is faithful. And if we look carefully at the stories of our past that are laced with betrayal, loss, and bitterness, we will find they are also marked by memories of his surprising protection.

—Dan Allender in THE HEALING PATH

---

19. How have you betrayed God?

20. How has God responded?

21. How does your experience of betrayal help you appreciate the loving way in which God has responded to you when you have betrayed him?

22. What would you like to say to God right now?

POWERLESSNESS AND THE LOSS OF HOPE

*A companion study to Chapter 5
in THE HEALING PATH*

In this session you will examine the dynamics of power-lessness. Unlike session 4, in which you reflected only on the past, this session will call you to reflect on both past and present situations in which you feel or felt powerless. When you look at the past, however, you may want to focus on one experience that made you feel profoundly powerless.

Powerlessness is the agony of being caught in a trap from which we can't extricate ourselves. We are naked, impotent, helpless, and without the resources, power, or friends to make the kind of difference we desire.

To be powerless does not mean we can't make decisions or respond to situations; rather, to be pow-erless is to be unable to erase the damage and paint the good we so deeply desire.... No, we aren't power-less to change, and yet we are powerless to escape the incessant struggle and the slow, slow progress of change.

—Dan Allender in THE HEALING PATH

---

1. In what current situations do you feel powerless to shape circumstances and protect yourself from suffering? (For example, you are not powerless to treat someone else with love, but you are powerless to make that person give you the love you want.)

2. In your list of situations under question 1, put a "W" beside those items in which the *world* (circumstances outside you) is the source of your powerlessness. Put an "F" beside those items in which you are powerless over your *flesh* (your own self-will, your instincts and natural inclinations that seem to have a mind of their own). Put a "D" beside any items where you think the *devil* (supernatural evil) is at work. You might have more than one letter beside some items.

At [times] the only way to break the bondage [of evil] is to give up everything that the comfort of the web provided. Evil knows we would rather delude ourselves, deny the truth, and eventually justify even harmful behavior as our only choice.

—Dan Allender in THE HEALING PATH

---

3. What is one past experience that made you feel profoundly powerless?

4. How were the world, the flesh, and/or the devil at work in that situation?

Martyrdom, or self-righteous suffering, sighs and finds satisfaction in its helplessness. No one can, no one could help. No one cares. No one understands, and so I will bear this suffering with no complaint, which means with no desire. The self-righteous martyr suffers alone, publicly....

Belligerence is the swaggering threat of violence. It is cocky and sure and is not concerned about addressing injustice; rather, it seeks to create chaos.... Most violence...is not justice based; it is an effort to restore pride and a sense of personal power through vengeance. Violence that stems from belligerence demeans and tears down in order to make someone pay....

The disengaged...do not use their powerlessness to make others feel powerless, as martyrs do, nor do they pull down the towers of power, as the belligerent; instead, the disengaged flee this world and fantasize about an annulment of their condition. The

fantasy of winning the lottery, of inheriting something of surprising value, of receiving a check in the
mail from an unknown patron wings many of us
above our common lot of suffering. The romance
novel, the soap opera, and the sports game serve as
an escape that takes away the consciousness of our
plight through a vicarious attachment to the dreams
and lives of others....

Each style of managing powerlessness is a flight
from hope. Powerlessness, like poverty, steals the passion to remember or dream.

—Dan Allender in THE HEALING PATH

5. In response to those experiences of powerlessness, is
it more typical for you to play the martyr, to be belligerent, or to disengage? (Or do you use more than
one of these strategies?)

6. How do you act out your martyrdom, belligerence,
or disengagement? Describe one way in which you
typically do this in a relationship.

Sacred discontent is not mere dissatisfaction that
turns the heart to complain and disengage. It is a
holy hunger to enter a heart or situation so that we
can offer incarnate love and know the same at the
roots of our soul....

Disengagement is a flight from risk. It is a refusal
to suffer any more losses. We would prefer to hunker
down, dull our desire, and drift into distractions that

take away our holy hunger for more. For many of us,
the meaning of our lives will not be found until we
risk moving out of our realm of safety.

—Dan Allender in THE HEALING PATH

During twenty-five years of tough ministry, the apostle
Paul became intimate with powerlessness. He was in and
out of jail, was beaten more than once, and got used to
being run out of town. He had powerful enemies.

Eventually, he spent several long years in prison—
and apparently in chains—awaiting a trial that never
seemed to come. During this wretched period he wrote a
remarkably cheerful letter to his friends in Philippi. The
believers in Philippi were also on a first-name basis with
powerlessness—their town was run by Roman army vet-
erans who viewed their religion with disgust.

Read Philippians 1:12-30 and 4:10-13.

7. As he writes this letter, in what ways is Paul powerless against the world, the flesh, and/or evil?

8. Does Paul sound like a martyr in this letter? What
   evidence for or against this do you see in the text?

9. What signs of sacred discontent with the status quo does Paul show?

10. Would you describe Paul more as belligerent or eagerly patient? What evidence do you find in his letter?

11. Did Paul disengage, or risk? How can you tell?

12. What do you think enabled Paul to deal with a powerless situation like this?

We all want to change, but change requires a herculean effort that seldom brings the immediate benefits needed to reinforce the initial cost and disruption change entails. The formula for change seems to be: High cost today—no gain for a long, long time; high gain in the distant future—*if* one perseveres daily in hope.

But the mounting remains of failures loom large against the horizon of hope. I failed with this diet. I failed in this relationship. I failed in this commitment. I failed in this project. I've failed enough! I don't care to fail again. I will only set forth to change myself when I absolutely must or when the prospect of success is nearly sure.

> What this means for many of us is a life of end-
> less repetition and a good but routine existence.
> —Dan Allender in THE HEALING PATH

13. In what ways (if any) does "endless repetition and a good but routine existence" describe your life?

14. When you think about the long process and high cost of changing what you can change in your life and your world, does sacred discontent motivate you to go for it? Or does the cost seem too high? What goes through your mind as you think about sacred discontent?

15. Look back at the situations you listed in question 1. Although you may be powerless to change the circumstances, the Holy Spirit does give you power to act within those circumstances, just as he gave Paul power.

    Choose one situation and describe what you do have the power to do. What would waiting and risking look like in that situation?

16. Take a minute to pray about this situation. Are you going to wait and risk, or are you going to settle for your pattern of martyrdom, belligerence, and/or disengagement?

AMBIVALENCE AND THE LOSS OF LOVE

*A companion study to Chapter 6
in THE HEALING PATH*

In this session you will look at ambivalence and its damaging effects: shame, dogmatism, acceptance of the status quo, a rule-bound life, an unwillingness to love passionately. You will also consider whether you want to take the healing path away from that damage. Once again, you will probably find it helpful to keep in mind a specific area of your life in which you experience ambivalence, whether that is something mundane like the decision to buy a house, or something profound like the decision to risk caring deeply for someone.

> Ambivalence is the emotional battle with two (or more) minds, wills, and desires. It is not being double-minded in the sense of being duplicitous or two-faced; rather, it is feeling two contrary energies moving us in opposite directions, being caught in the bind of opposing desires, feeling divided and torn.
>
> —Dan Allender in THE HEALING PATH

1. Describe an area of your life in which you are ambivalent, in which you feel torn between two or more opposing desires. Tell what those conflicting

desires are (or tell what you want to do and what you think you should do).

2. To what is this area of ambivalence linked? Check all that apply.
   ☐ a fulfilled dream that falls short of your expectations
   ☐ a gift that makes you feel needed, but perhaps also used
   ☐ suffering
   ☐ abuse
   ☐ none of the above

God gives us the frightening freedom to find our own way after naming the path of following him. He points us toward the way and then lets us discover him through our missteps and our successes. Freedom deepens and does not ease ambivalence.

—Dan Allender in THE HEALING PATH

---

3. When you think about the ambivalence in your life, what do you want God to do? (For instance, do you want God to tell you what to do? Fan the flames of faith, hope, and love inside you? Help you understand the spiritual implications of your options? Give you courage?)

It is exhausting to be caught in the throes of ambivalence. To not know the "right" thing to do (or even
to know it while being drawn to the alternative) is to
feel drained and overwhelmed by indecision and
ambiguity. One way out is to muster arrogant confidence, the certainty of dogmatic conviction: This is
the *right* and *only* decision. To maintain this perspec-
tive is exhausting as well. Dogmatism requires a level
of arrogance that is like carrying an extra thirty
pounds in a pack. It can be done, but it slows the
carrier's pace and hampers movement.... [Further,
dogmatism] compels us to push others to be and do
what makes us comfortable, rather than allowing
them to join in the process. Ambivalence often creates a dogmatic, pushy heart that violates love.

—Dan Allender in THE HEALING PATH

4. When you read the above description of dogmatism, to what extent does it sound like you? In what
   areas of life (if any) do you tend toward dogmatism?

5. Do you tend to escape ambivalence by settling for
   the status quo but not letting yourself think or feel
   about the alternatives? In what areas of life (if any)
   do you do this?

As the number of rules increases, the possibility of being in a position where one doesn't know what to do decreases. Most people are more comfortable in a rule-driven culture where behavior is prescribed and uncertainty largely eliminated. The resulting loss of freedom is rewarded with a greater distance from the prospect of shame. Such striving to avoid ambivalence and shame is the motivating force that shapes the soul of a Pharisee and the culture of legalism.
—Dan Allender in THE HEALING PATH

6. In what areas of life do you like knowing what the rules are?

7. To what extent do you think your attitude toward rules is influenced by a fear of making a decision that will shame you in front of others?

Ambivalence grows to the degree we are unaware of its driving source of shame....

Shame comes when an accusation exposes our dark inner world to others. Shame makes us feel unlovable and unable to love. Most of us make our inner world off-limits to even our most intimate companions or spouse, because to open our heart is to reveal the confusion, disgust, arousal, and shame within. Instead, we wear a guise of normalcy, a veneer of acceptability—a mask that keeps relationships in place but leaves the heart alone.

—Dan Allender in THE HEALING PATH

8. On a separate sheet of paper, write down three things that you don't want anyone to know about you: things you've done; things you think about; qualities, habits, or secrets. You can tear up this sheet when you're finished with this session, and you don't have to tell anyone what you wrote.

9. What do you fear would happen if people knew those things about you?

10. Is there a connection between any of these three things and the area of ambivalence you described in question 1? If so, what's the connection? (You can write on your separate sheet of paper if you're concerned about privacy.)

11. Are you ever ashamed of longing for deep, passionate love? If so, what seems shameful about that?

12. How does shame hinder you from loving people deeply and well?

Ambivalence can lead to a jaded, cynical view of
love. Love is work; it pays little and requires everything.… A passionate connection to a person that
ultimately leads to the sacrifice of one's own identity
and safety is viewed by the self-righteous as senseless,
sick, and codependent.

—Dan Allender in THE HEALING PATH

Crucifixion was the most shameful means of death
known in either the Roman or Jewish worlds. The
Romans reserved it for slaves and scum. The Jews associ-
ated it with Deuteronomy 21:22-23, which stated that
"anyone who is hung on a tree is under God's curse."
From the moment of his arrest until his death, Jesus was
subjected to one public humiliation after another.

Read Matthew 26:59-75 and 27:11-50.

13. List all the ways in which Jesus was shamed at his
    trial and crucifixion.

14. Why was Jesus willing to endure all this shame?

15. Jesus wasn't ashamed to express his anguish at being
    cut off from the Father's love while he bore the
    curse of the Cross (Matthew 27:46). In fact, God
    wasn't ashamed to make the Cross a flagrant, public
    display of his desire to be loved by us. If God isn't
    ashamed that the whole cosmos knows how much

44

he wants to be loved, what difference does that make to your answer to question 11?

Before his arrest, Jesus struggled with ambivalence. At Gethsemane, he wrestled between his desire to do his Father's will and his desire to avoid the ordeal of the Cross (Matthew 26:36-46). Yet Jesus neither sidestepped his ambivalence nor allowed it to paralyze him. Nor did he allow shame to keep him from acting with passionate love toward God and humans.

16. What do you think enabled Jesus to continue to love and not be shut down by shame?

17. Think about the areas of shame you listed in question 8. Consider them in light of Jesus' shame. What thoughts or emotions come to mind as you put the two side by side?

18. What do you think Jesus would say to you about the area of ambivalence you named in question 1?

If you are meeting with a group, read together the introduction to session 7 of this study guide. It contains instructions for a group exercise for which you will need to plan ahead if you decide to do it. A group is an excellent place for people to reflect together on the core themes of one another's lives.

THE WAGER OF FAITH

A companion study to Chapter 7
in THE HEALING PATH

In this session you will look at the roles of memory and story in shaping our doubt and our faith. You will look at two stories from your own past—one of harm and betrayal, and one of redemption—to see how these stories have affected the person you have become.

If you are meeting with a group, you may find it helpful to begin this session by letting each person share briefly how it has felt to dig into his or her stories throughout this study.

One of the important concepts of chapter 7 is how stories reveal the core themes of our lives. It is often easier for other people to see the connections between our stories and our themes than it is for us. Hence, a group is an excellent setting for generous, nonintrusive reflection about one's life. If you agree to do so as a group, take some time before your meeting to think about the stories you have heard from the other members. Jot some notes about the themes you have heard from each person. Questions 5, 6, 8, and 18 in this session may spark your thinking. Focus on encouraging and building each other up rather than on being critical. Write notes for each person on a separate index card or sheet of paper. In this way, you can give your notes to the people after your discussion.

Question 18 invites you to discuss the connections you sense in each other's stories. Such a discussion could take quite a bit of time, but it would be extremely valuable. No one should be required to be the focus of this discussion; rather, each member should have the opportunity to ask for the group's impressions if they're wanted.

My faith in God's character grows to the degree I remember God. Faith is trust in the goodness of God. I grow as I recall and recollect the stories of God in the Bible, in the lives of others, and in my own life. To recall is to name, with sufficient detail to be moved by God's presence, the life scenes or events in which he showed up as Rescuer. The external world and our internal gyroscope are never so clear that we have absolute assurance that a personal God is at work redeeming us. Instead, we have a gallery of pictures—a wall of remembrance that holds the faces of the actors in our lives who spoke their part in the play of our redemption.

—Dan Allender in THE HEALING PATH

---

1. Why does Dr. Allender think memory is the key to faith?

Every person alive has legions of stories of heartache and shame, loneliness and betrayal. But every human being also has at least one story of redemption that is full of surprise and delight.... It is in that one story

(and likely many more) that we can't deny or forget
that God wooed us to the desert to redeem us. The
process is not easy or mechanical, but the healing path
of remembering our stories points toward God's incon-
ceivable, slow-moving, strange plan of redemption.

—Dan Allender in THE HEALING PATH

2. Tell one story from your past in which God rescued
or redeemed you.

3. How easy was it for you to recall a story of redemption? Why do you suppose that's the case?

In a tragic and wonderful sense, it is suspense and
drama that brings out the reality of what is in our
hearts. The people of God are pushed against the
Red Sea, and when their backs are against the wall,
they turn against God. Drama reveals. It exposes us
and allows the work of God to proceed in our lives.

—Dan Allender in THE HEALING PATH

4. In earlier sessions of this study you told stories of
your experiences of betrayal, powerlessness, and

ambivalence. Choose one of those stories and describe how it has affected the person you have become.

Few people have a list of the scenes that have shaped their lives. Fewer still have written out the scenes in narrative fashion. And even fewer have even asked the question, "What are the themes of my stories?" It is not enough to ask, "What is God trying to teach me?"; far more, we must ask, "What does God want me to become?" We get a glimpse of the answer only by considering the themes of our stories.

To discover our themes, we must listen to the core stories of our lives. We must listen in the same way we embrace a friend: with open arms, waiting, anticipating, holding, and then letting go. It is not something done in a day; it is a lifelong process. But in calling forth our core stories, we must also participate in the ordering of them. Themes don't smack us in the face when we look for them; instead, we must actively arrange, rearrange, and create the order that makes most sense at any given point in our lives.

—Dan Allender in THE HEALING PATH

---

5. What is the theme of the redemptive story you recounted in question 2? (That is, "This story is about....")

6. What is the theme of the story of harm you recalled in question 4?

7. In Luke 17:1-6, Jesus says that the one who betrayed you deserves drowning, while at the same time he calls you to forgive if there is repentance. What would it look like for you to forgive this wrong without minimizing its harm?

8. From what you can see of the way God has worked through your story so far, what does God want you to become?

The wager of faith is simple: Which stories will win my heart?… The wager is won only when even the smallest story of redemption means more to us than the greatest betrayal and loss….

What then is faith? It is the childlike wonder in a story so good it can't be true, but deep down to our toes we know if it is not true then we don't exist.

—Dan Allender in THE HEALING PATH

Psalm 22 is one of two psalms that Jesus quoted while he hung on the cross. The gospels record him saying only the first verse, but they allude to Psalm 22 several times in their depictions of the Crucifixion.

In the first eleven verses of this psalm, the poet goes back and forth in his mind between faith and doubt. In verses 1-2 he expresses his desperation, then in verses 3-5 he reminds himself, "Yet...." Again, in verses 6-8 he says, "But...," and in verses 9-11 he answers, "Yet...."

Read Psalm 22:1-11. You might want to read the whole psalm to get a sense of how it ends.

9. In verses 1 and 2, how does the psalmist express his doubts about God?

10. In what ways, if any, can you identify with the psalmist's feelings in these two verses?

11. In verses 3-5, the psalmist shifts to remind himself of some things he knows. Of what does he remind himself?

12. Why do you think he reminds himself of these things?

13. How would you summarize his feelings in verses 6-8?

14. He turns back to memory again in verses 9-10. Of what does he remind himself this time?

15. Why do you suppose Jesus chose this psalm to recite while hanging on the cross?

This psalmist knows the stories of how his fathers and mothers in faith have trusted in God and have not been disappointed (verse 5). One difficulty many of us have today is that we don't know these stories, so we can't bring them to mind when we need them. There is much to be gained in reading these stories, both those in the Bible and those about men and women who have lived in faith since the Bible was written. If you're not familiar with Exodus 1–15, Mark 14–16, and the book of Acts, those are good places to begin.

16. Look ahead to the next six months of your healing path. How can you take advantage of the biblical stories to build your faith? What is something specific and concrete you can do?

17. During the next six months, how can you begin searching out the themes of your story?

18. If you are meeting with a group, ask the group what connections they see between the stories you have told them and the core themes of your life.

THE DREAM OF HOPE

A companion study to Chapter 8
in THE HEALING PATH

In this session you will reflect on your ability to desire and hope for the future. If you are meeting as a group, you might want to do the imagination exercise in question 6 together. The leader can read the biblical text and the instructions while the other group members sit with their eyes closed. Allow at least two or three minutes of silence. Afterward, discuss how it felt to do this.

Be aware that talking about dreams for the future requires more risk than does talking about the past. People hold dreams close to their hearts, and even if they admit their deepest desires to themselves, they may never have admitted them to someone else. Think about what you can do to make the group a safe place in which to dream together.

> When the storms come, we typically respond to them by raging against the gale or turning away from the loss, resigned and despondent. Most choose the latter option, because once we relinquish desire the loss does not seem so severe. But resignation is always a betrayal, not only of desire but also of hope....
>
> Biblical hope is substantial faith regarding the future. Hope looks at the shattered remnants of the

soul hit by the storm and envisions not merely
rebuilding, but rebuilding a life that has even more
purpose and meaning than existed before the loss.

—Dan Allender in THE HEALING PATH

1. When something painful happens to you, are you
more likely to rage or resign yourself to the circumstances? Describe your typical response.

2. Which of the following do you desire most intensely?
   - ☐ passionate sexual union
   - ☐ sumptuous food
   - ☐ justice between you and your enemies
   - ☐ other: _____
   - ☐ nothing

3. Would you describe yourself as a person with strong
desires? Explain.

4. What's the difference between hope and fantasy?

Think of the finest meal you've ever eaten. Recall the
most pleasurable sexual moment with your beloved.
Then realize that your memory offers but a glimmer

of the glory that awaits you. Hope grows only to the degree that the pleasures of this world serve as a window to the glory of the next....

There is an ancient language in us, a memory from Eden that resounds in us as we recall our past and read about the promises of our future. Hope is leaning into the unknown, risking our lives for a future that is promised in the Word and tasted in a few hors d'oeuvres from our story. We are meant to sensualize heaven, not spiritualize it with images that bore us to tears.

—Dan Allender in THE HEALING PATH

5. What do you think about this idea of the pleasures of this world serving as a window to the glory of the next? (You might look at Romans 1:20. How is God's divine nature revealed in chocolate cake?)

Most of us find it difficult to yield ourselves to the biblical images of what Dr. Allender calls "the far future" and Jesus called "the kingdom of God" or "the kingdom of the heavens." The biblical images are such sensualized poetry that we may find them raw and embarrassing. We tend to think of heaven as an airy, sedate place or a spiritual realm, not as a place of feasting, drinking, and laughter with animals everywhere. However, the image of the future as a feast echoes from the prophets to the gospels to Revelation.

Read Isaiah 25:6-12 aloud to yourself. Then go back and reread just the first sentence. You might read it a couple of times until you really hear it.

6. Imagine yourself at a huge table. It's covered with your favorite foods, as well as other delicacies you've never tried before. At your elbow is a glass of something wonderful to drink. On either side of you are your two closest friends in the world, perhaps people from your childhood whom you haven't seen in years. Across the table are people from the past—saints whom you've always wanted to talk to. As you look up and down the table you see people you've missed and people you'd hate to miss. To your astonishment, there are also people whom you never thought you'd see here. All of these people are eating, drinking, talking, laughing, and asking questions to get to know you. Even the saints seem to be enjoying what you have to say. At the head of the table sits Jesus, listening closely to a child chatting next to him. Every now and again he sends a wink your way.

Now close your eyes. Take a few minutes to let this scene sink in. Mentally fill in the details. Who are the people at your right and your left? Who sits across from you? What food is on the table? What are you feeling?

7. Open your eyes. What was it like to let your imagination dwell on a biblical text like that? What thoughts and emotions came up?

8. Perhaps a noisy party isn't your idea of a good time. If not, what would be your ideal image of heaven?

9. What's the benefit of letting ourselves dwell on images of the far future?

10. How comfortable are you with desiring, dreaming, and hoping? Why do you suppose that is?

Sin and its effects cannot be eradicated, but redemption can bring an even greater strength to a relationship or a heart than existed before. The scars of sin and death can't be erased, but they can become the weather-beaten marks of character that bring depth and intrigue to what would have been merely a beautiful but ordinary vase. God's passion is to weave glory out of the broken shards of past sexual abuse, an affair, financial disaster, a divorce, death, or any other experience of powerlessness or sin.

—Dan Allender in THE HEALING PATH

---

11. What do you most hope for yourself in this life?

12. What is hard for you about hoping, or about acknowledging your hopes to others?

Hope is solid and sure, but only for the final outcome. It grows only to the degree we lean into the unknown and risk the present for the sake of the future....

Hope is not docile, anemic patience that serenely waits with hands folded and eyes closed. Instead, hope cries to God in despair and protest. Job knocks on God's door until he answers. Hope cries out for God to turn from his silence and speak....

Hope is not an absence of sorrow but a refusal to allow powerlessness to silence our cry or to shake our confidence in God. Instead, we are to call on God to be God—to protest his silence and anticipate the day when he speaks.

—Dan Allender in THE HEALING PATH

---

13. What do you think God is calling you to risk?

14. Are you more likely to pray crying out to God or with hands folded and eyes closed? Why is that?

15. If you were going to cry out to God, protesting his silence, what would you say? (You might just say it, preferably aloud. Find someplace where you won't worry about being overheard, and tell God what you really think.)

Surrender confesses that our deepest desire is not to succeed in business, to marry, to have kids, to be well or simply happy; instead, our deepest hunger is *to see him*. Surrender goes even further: It despises anything and everything in us and outside of us that compromises our passion to be caught up in his glory and love....

As we surrender our imaginations to a future glory, we are not recasting the present in terms of how we want the world to be (that is illusion), nor are we reordering our lives to add new elements and delete the ones we don't want (that is delusion). Instead, surrender is holding reality firm in the grip of unflinching honesty while also seeing every moment in the light of the invisible, eternal, and redeemed. It is the visionary gift of the interior decorator who can come into a dilapidated room and see new form, color, and structure.

—Dan Allender in THE HEALING PATH

---

16. In session 7 you thought about what God wants you to become. As you've reflected on the glory ahead of you and told God what you most desire, what more have you learned about what God wants you to become?

THE DANCE OF LOVE

A companion study to Chapter 9
in THE HEALING PATH

In this session you will consider the choice between loving and closing your heart—from remembered love (past) to dreamt love (future) to loving in the present moment.

Love requires faith, but remembering puts us in a bind. After all, not all our memories of love are "North Stars" that guide us confidently into the future. The memories that sting most are those that remind us of love that led to shame. Shame is the exposure of our foolishness to have trusted that another person would be true and good toward us. If we give that person our heart and then are betrayed, we have nothing and are no thing. We are no one. We lose face. It is losing face that most deeply provokes shame. All of us have memories of romantic, filial, professional, and ministry relationships in which we have lost face.

The memories create a dilemma as to which story, which face, we will allow to define us. We can't answer the call to love unless we adore the faces of others. We can't love without potentially losing face ourselves. We can't love unless we remember the faces in our lives that have been our bridge to God.

61

But in remembering we also recall faces that have
scorned, used, and betrayed us.

—Dan Allender in THE HEALING PATH

1. Whose are some of the faces that have loved you in
   the past?

2. Whose are some of the faces that have shamed you?

3. To this point in your life, which of these faces have
   you allowed to define you?

There is a door to every heart. And every experience
in life is either invited in or turned away. It is impossi-
ble to describe the door or say it is a mere metaphor.
We take in or we turn away. We hear the knock, or we
ignore the noise and turn our attention more deliber-
ately to other stimuli. The decision to hear a knock
and open the door is a moral stance that determines
how much we are willing to change and grow.

—Dan Allender in THE HEALING PATH

4. When did you last hear God knocking at the door of your heart, inviting you to love and be loved? What did you do?

I'm troubled to think how often I enter an evening meal with my family, or watch the evening news, or read a book in the same frame of mind. Am I awake? Is my heart open to hear the people who have a claim on my heart?

Gabriel Marcel said that availability is a "receptiveness to the abundance of the world." The world is fragrant with the glory of God, often hidden and frequently intertwined with the strange and unexpected. The abundance is present, nevertheless, in the twinkling of nearly every moment. "It is the ability to abandon oneself to whatever one encounters… to transform mere circumstances into 'occasions' or indeed into opportune situations. It is to contribute to the shaping of one's fate by impressing one's own distinctive mark upon it."[1]

"Response-ability," then, is my capacity to hear the call of abundance (or the lack thereof) and pledge myself to the good of others in that moment.

—Dan Allender in THE HEALING PATH

---

[1] Gabriel Marcel, *Homo Viator* (Gloucester, Mass.: Peter Smith Publisher, 1978), 187.

5. Think about your most recent encounter with one or more people. How present and available were you? How did you (or didn't you) show yourself to be present, available, and pledged to others' good in that moment?

6. What would it have looked like and felt like for you to be abundantly present in love in that situation?

Waiting requires the discipline to set aside short-term pleasure or quick satisfaction for a greater fulfillment. Waiting is sustained by the anticipation of fullness; therefore, it is sustained by dreaming.

A believing heart dreams through prayer. Waiting does not mean sitting. It means kneeling, submitting, and humbling myself not only to the expanse of dreams desired, but to the acknowledgment that I can't make the dream appear. Dreams that involve the depths of what my soul desires are utterly outside the realm of my control....

Jesus invites familiarity and urgency. Far more, he invites desperate, bold prayer. Many pray with a perfunctory, soulless recitation of magic words, sincerely said but robotically offered. It is not dissimilar from flight attendants who read the information required by the FAA in order for a flight to take off.

It's good information that most people ignore,
including the one reading/praying it.

Bold, naked prayer leaves us between God's
promise and absence, between a divine rock and a
hard place. On one hand is the sure promise of his
love, on the other is his silence or apparent inactivity.
The waiting continues. I cry out: Redeem me.
Change me. Heal me. The tears flow and my heart
beats fast in anticipation of the dream fulfilled. I
open my eyes and the room has not changed, the
clouds have not parted, and my soul often feels more
empty and alone than it did before I prayed.

—Dan Allender in THE HEALING PATH

7. In the situation you discussed in questions 5 and 6,
   perhaps you were not the abundantly loving person
   you desire to be. Reflect on Dr. Allender's words
   about waiting, dreaming, and praying. Then write a
   prayer that expresses your deepest desire for the
   kind of person you want to be in your relationships.

8. How easy is desperate, bold prayer for you? Why do
   you suppose that's the case?

9. Dr. Allender urges us to "hate deadness more than shame." At this point in your journey, which do you hate more: deadness or shame? How does that choice play itself out in your relationships?

The Song of Songs is a dramatic poem composed for the wedding of King Solomon. It's about 2,500 years older than *Romeo and Juliet,* and it's proof that nobody writes a love scene better than God. Through erotic, sensual dialogue, the bride and bridegroom express their desire for each other.

The Song is perhaps best understood in layers: it really is about the passion between a man and a woman, but their passion becomes a window into the love between God and mortals. The poem's climax is the bride's wedding vow. In the excerpt below, the ancient "seal" serves roughly the same purpose as the wedding ring—an outward seal or pledge of the heart's commitment. Read the excerpt aloud as though you are reading it to your beloved.

> Set me as a seal upon your heart,
>   as a seal upon your arm;
> for love is strong as death,
>   passion fierce as the grave.
> Its flashes are flashes of fire,
>   a raging flame.
> Many waters cannot quench love,
>   neither can floods drown it.
> If one offered for love
>   all the wealth of one's house,
>   it would be utterly scorned.
>   (Song of Songs 8:6-7, NRSV)

10. Do you believe love is strong as death? What makes you believe or disbelieve?

11. Think about God saying these words to you, loving you with this passion. How do you reply to God?

12. We usually think of unquenchable passion as the essence of romantic love, not for love between long-married people, parents and their aloof teenager, or members of a church. Yet why is unquenchable passion necessary in all our efforts to love?

13. Imagine loving the people you wrote about in questions 5 and 6 with unquenchable passion. What would it take for that to be possible for you?

Love lets go of its inalienable rights; it leaves others free to respond to or reject it. Love does not grasp and hold on to others, compelling them to live for us. We care for, provide for, instruct, and rear our children. And then they leave. The same model applies in mentoring relationships. Each person we encounter is a being we are meant to bless and serve. Each person is meant in some way to bless and serve us, or the lack of mutuality will strip the relationship of truth and depth. The intertwining of hearts nourishes and grows courage to walk further on the long healing journey.

—Dan Allender in THE HEALING PATH

14. How does knowing people will eventually leave you affect your ability to love them passionately? (You might have a particular relationship in mind as you think about this.)

15. How would your life be different if you truly believed that nothing and no one but God could satisfy your longing to love someone passionately?

If you are meeting with a group, close by talking about how the group has blessed and served you.

Living a Radical Life

A companion study to Chapter 10
in The Healing Path

In this session you will consider the question, "Why am I here?" You won't be able to answer the question fully and finally, but you will get a sense of how to go about seeking an answer. Dr. Allender speaks of becoming more unique and more like Jesus through intrigue, imagination, and incarnate care of others; and through disturbing, drawing, and directing others toward God.

Begin by looking at an encounter among Jesus, a stranger, and Jesus' friends. Read Mark 10:17-31.

1. This encounter begins as the stranger runs up to Jesus and falls on his knees. He asks the kind of profound question most of us would love to be asked: "Good teacher, what must I do to inherit eternal life?"

   If someone asked you this, what do you think you would probably say and/or do?

2. How is Jesus' response to the man like or unlike what you would do or say in a similar situation?

3. In response to the man, Jesus questions the man's respectful use of the word *good*. (Does that seem a bit rude?) Then he lists five of the Ten Commandments. He omits the four commandments about worshiping God above all other gods, as well as the one about coveting one's neighbor's possessions. (You can compare Jesus' list of commandments to the full list in Exodus 20:1-17.)

   What do you think Jesus is trying to accomplish by responding like this?

4. The man asserts he has kept all five commandments since he was a boy. How would you probably respond if someone said that to you?   ·

5. How is Jesus' response like or unlike what you would say?

6. What is Jesus' heartfelt attitude toward this man? How is it like or unlike the way you would feel about such a man?

7. In the end, the man leaves in great sadness. Do you think Jesus regarded the encounter as a failure? What makes you say that?

8. As the story goes on, it shifts into a conversation between Jesus and his disciples. What emotional reactions do they have to Jesus' statements in verse 24, and again in verse 26?

9. What can we learn from this episode about how to interact with people?

We must move into a world that will be intrigued with us only if we live surprising, compelling lives that offer more than can be found in other stories and communities. Our calling is to be in the world without living according to the elemental principles, the core assumptions, of a fallen order. We are to be in the world, to incarnate the gospel in the flesh of our stories and struggles.

—Dan Allender in THE HEALING PATH

---

10. In a typical week, what sorts of interactions do you have with non-Christians?

11. Do you believe it's possible for you to live a surprising, compelling life that offers more than can be found in the stories of the world? What leads you to believe or disbelieve this?

12. Many of us feel we're too busy either surviving or healing to be deeply involved in the lives of people outside our immediate circle of family and friends. However, most of us already have at least a few people in our paths for whom we can be the presence of Jesus. Make a list of people you already encounter (people at your job or your kids' schools, someone who does work around your home, and so on) who need to have God made flesh in their lives.

> Few people are intrigued by others. Few people fol-
> low up conversation with an invitation for others to
> tell their stories. We are rarely curious about each
> other's individual tastes, convictions, and interests,
> let alone the stories that provide the thematic struc-
> ture to our lives.
>
> —Dan Allender in THE HEALING PATH

13. What tends to be your attitude toward new people
    you meet? Are you curious and intrigued?

14. Do the people you've known for a long time
    intrigue you? Why do you suppose that's the case?

15. What could build your sense of curiosity about
    people?

> Our calling is to be more in awe of, more willing to
> risk entry into the stories of others. But when we
> enter we are not human if we merely listen and ask
> questions; we must imagine and speak to the dream
> of glory. To be human is to see what can't be seen, to
> give ourselves to the future through the labor pains
> of creative struggle....
>
> "So we fix our eyes not on what is seen, but on
> what is unseen. For what is seen is temporary, but
> what is unseen is eternal" (2 Corinthians 4:18). Using

73

our imagination to see the unseen gives up convention
and the-way-it-has-always-been-done to see what has
yet to be revealed. If the imagining is of God, it leads
not merely to gratitude but to a passionate desire to
draw out the glory of those in our care.

—Dan Allender in THE HEALING PATH

16. As you look back over your life, who have been the
people who saw and drew forth from within you
the person they imagined you could be? How did
they do this?

17. Think of someone important to you. What do you
see in that person that could be but isn't yet?

Speaking truth in love is simple and requires our
very life and soul. More often than not it is merely
saying to the emperor, "You are buck naked. Where
are your clothes?" It is not difficult to see areas of
failure in others, but it requires a kindness and a
depth of participation that may cost us the relationship if we speak. The difficulty is rarely in knowing
what to say, but in saying it with a heart that grieves
for the other's pain and depravity and dreams for
their freedom and glory.

—Dan Allender in THE HEALING PATH

18. In his encounter with the rich man, how did Jesus do what Dr. Allender describes in the paragraph above?

19. What would you like to say to the person you considered in question 17? What questions could you ask to expose that person's heart? Or what truth could you speak?

20. Do you grieve for that person's pain and depravity and dream for their freedom and glory? Or are you more annoyed, frustrated, or hurt by their depravity?

21. Take a minute to write a prayer that expresses grief and dreaming for that person.

> [God] has given us our unique set of stories to make something known about himself, something that reveals his infinitely variegated being. We must follow the path of our personal redemption to understand the calling that we alone can answer.
>
> —Dan Allender in THE HEALING PATH

22. What is one thing about God that your story makes known?

> To respond to our individual calling is to live out the themes of our stories—themes that fill us with sorrow, anger, pleasure, and joy—for God's glory. God has crafted each of us with burdens we can't escape....
>
> A burden is a passion that typically arises from the mesh of our story. As a result, to neglect our burden is to lose our soul.... What are the themes of your story? Where does your heart break with sorrow for what is still unredeemed? What arouses your anger when you see evil score another victory? What brings a *yes!* to your soul when you give?
>
> —Dan Allender in THE HEALING PATH

23. What is one of your burdens? If you don't know, how can you begin to find out?

24. Being intrigued with people is a habit that we have
    to cultivate, if it doesn't come to us naturally. Every-
    one is interesting if we know how to see them.
    Look for a chance this week to show real interest in
    learning someone's story.

If you're meeting with a group, you may want to treat the
Bible study (questions 1 through 9) as background and
focus your discussion on a few of the other questions.
Also, talk about the things that seem to hinder you from
being deeply involved in people's lives. Perhaps your
obstacle is busyness, fear, or the sense of being one lone
person who is just beginning to get a grip on your own
life. You may find that you can overcome these obstacles
by teaming up. Perhaps the most surprising, compelling
aspect of your life that you can show to outsiders is the
way in which the members of your group care for each
other. Is there someone you can invite to join you? Can
you throw a party and invite neighbors as well as your
friends from your group? Is there something creative you
can do together for your community, like the dog wash by
the Bainbridge Island church described in the book?

Dream together. How can you team up to intrigue
the people around you?

INVITING OTHERS TO LIVE

A companion study to Chapter 11
in THE HEALING PATH

In this session you will explore the art of redemptive conversation. It sounds tricky: present to past, past to future, future to present, present to eternity—what is all that? Hence, you will focus on the concrete example of the airplane conversation. But more important than the details of technique is the foundational question, "Do I have what it takes to do this?" You will consider this question in light of some words from 2 Corinthians.

A person who lives a radical life,…who is on the healing path toward becoming more fully himself and more essentially like Jesus, moves into the hearts of others with a redemptive purpose: to expose depravity and draw forth dignity. We are all a mixture of dignity (that which deeply desires what is good, lovely, and true) and depravity (that which refuses to confess that God is the sole good, beauty, and truth that our heart was made to desire—Psalm 73:25). Redemptive conversation delights in all that reflects dignity and disrupts whatever reeks of depravity. A radical life hears stories deeply enough to become a participant in another's life, an actor in a new story that God is telling on behalf of us all.

—Dan Allender in THE HEALING PATH

---

1. When you think about having redemptive conversa-
    tions with people, where would you place yourself
    on the following scale?

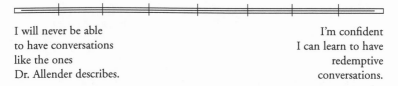

I will never be able   I'm confident
to have conversations   I can learn to have
like the ones   redemptive
Dr. Allender describes.   conversations.

2. What reasons lie behind your response to question 1?

It's tempting to leave redemptive conversation to the
experts—people like Dr. Allender who have years of train-
ing as counselors—or to the specially gifted, such as evan-
gelists and pastors. Jesus did not leave us out, however. He
turned over his ministry to his first followers and told them
to train the rest of us to do it too. Even someone as extra-
ordinary as the apostle Paul never lost sight of where his
capacity for ministry came from. In 2 Corinthians, he
spent a good deal of time boasting of his inadequacy in
order to illuminate the source of his confidence.

Read 2 Corinthians 3:18–4:11.

3. Consider 2 Corinthians 3:18. Is this true of you?
    What evidence can you begin to see?

4. In 4:3-4 and 8-11, how does Paul describe the difficult circumstances under which he engages in what Dr. Allender calls "the battle against evil's hatred of glory"?

5. What do you think Paul means when he refers to us as "jars of clay" (4:7)?

6. Why doesn't Paul lose heart when he contemplates the intense opposition from evil and his own mind and feet of clay?

   a. 4:1

   b. 4:5

   c. 4:6

   d. 4:7-11

7. Does any of this help build your courage to attempt redemptive conversations? If so, what in Paul's words do you find helpful? If not, what do you think is missing for you?

8. Perhaps the greatest barrier to our actually attempting redemptive conversations is shame: the fear of being exposed and rejected as inadequate, uninvited intruders into someone's private life. What do you think Paul would say to one who feared being shamed by failing in a redemptive conversation?

People in pain want to talk. They are very forgiving of our errors as long as we are neither pushy nor arrogant. We can bumble and learn. The reward is enormous.
—Dan Allender in THE HEALING PATH

9. Do you believe people in pain want to talk to you and will forgive your errors? What leads you to your belief?

FROM THE PRESENT TO THE PAST

The task required for redemptive conversation in the present is to look for a door, any door, that takes one from superficial data to matters of the heart. One of the best ways to find the door is to notice how the person draws you in or keeps you at a distance. The people who draw you in often fear loneliness more

than shame. Those who keep you at a distance usually fear shame more than loneliness. Most people will
draw and distance simultaneously. To find a door
that might be entered, all one needs to do is not
"give in" to the unstated instructions the person's
style dictates.

—Dan Allender in THE HEALING PATH

10. Read Dr. Allender's story of his conversation with
the electrical engineer (pages 215–234 in *The Healing Path*). What questions did he ask the man in
order to find doors to his heart?

11. What about these questions made them more effec-
tive at gently getting at the man's heart than the
typical questions people ask? What do you notice
about these questions that impresses you?

Curiosity and vulnerability are our best tools for
entering a person's heart. Once the door is open then
one must find the "tension point" or plot that is the
current matter of concern to the other....

There are gaps in every story. A gap is an unfin-
ished bridge between two elements in a person's story
that is probably significant to the development of a
plot. A person may not tell it because he views it as
incidental—or because it is too important. One will
never know until the gap is entered....

Past betrayal, powerlessness, and shame are the
formative, shaping influences that give direction to
our flight from God. If I want to move into matters
of faith, hope, and love, then I must enter a person's
past stories.

—Dan Allender in THE HEALING PATH

12. If a person wanted to draw out your passion—the
    things that really matter to your heart—what sorts
    of questions might he or she ask you? Think of
    questions that aren't excessively intrusive, such as,
    "What kind of art were you involved in?"

FROM THE PAST TO THE FUTURE

The past is the place we developed our deepest convictions about ourselves, life, and God. One cannot
enter another's past merely by hearing the conclu-
sions and convictions that resulted from it, but by
being invited into the story itself. To enter the past

one must ask permission. These life-shaping and raw scenes of life ought not be entered without invitation. When one is permitted into this terrain, the guest stands on holy ground....

The goal of redemptive conversation is not merely to move air or kill time, but to comprehend what the other loves. We all love someone or something. Resistance arises when we get too close to the scenes of the past that deeply matter.... Our response to resistance should be to draw forth its implications by connecting two points in a story and coming to a sum factor. Implications ought to be stated tentatively with ample room to differ, clarify, or add more data....

If the storyteller embraces the [implications], then it may be possible for the listener to move him from how he has attempted to make his life work (faith) to a vision of glory (hope) that could become a dream greater than the way he is living now.

—Dan Allender in THE HEALING PATH

13. In the airplane conversation, how did Dr. Allender...

a. ask permission to hear a life-shaping story from the engineer's past?

b. identify what the man desired and loved?

c. encounter resistance?

d. draw forth the implications of the pattern he was seeing in the man's story?

e. give the man a vision for a dream that would be greater than his current life?

FROM THE FUTURE
TO THE PRESENT

14. Why did Dr. Allender insist that the man ask him for a book?

FROM THE PRESENT TO ETERNITY

Discernment requires us to summarize our life themes through the use of at least one dramatic scene. My seatmate's life theme was connected to the brush-destruction scene. He would not want nor ask for anything; instead, he lived an indifferent, closed life of duty—he was an unbelieving older brother (Luke 15). My summary of his life-defining theme and its relationship to his marriage, parenting, and work created a dramatic moment for him in the present: *Now what?*

85

As simple as it is to say, few people ask others, "Now what?" In order to yield fruit, conversation must invite the other to discard the life themes that rob him of joy; it must direct him to the provision offered through the Cross. Movement toward eternity usually involves decisions that bring the heart to a crossroads.

—Dan Allender in THE HEALING PATH

15. How did Dr. Allender ask his seatmate, "Now what?"

16. Think of one or more persons in your life with whom you would like to have redemptive conversations. Take a few minutes to pray for those relationships. Ask God to give you the grace to see doors to their hearts—curious but non-intrusive questions that would begin to get at what goes on in their hearts.

Pray for ways to draw out their passions—the things that matter deeply to them. Pray for the privilege of being invited into one of their key stories from the past. Pray for the insight to perceive the connections between their stories and the themes of their lives. Pray for the people themselves, that God would work in their lives to soften their hearts to his presence. Ask God to give you a tender heart to care for and respect these people as you move redemptively into their lives. Finally, ask God to give you the courage to move redemptively into all your encounters with people during the coming week.

CREATING A COMMUNITY OF SOJOURNERS

A companion study to Chapter 12
in THE HEALING PATH

This session invites you to dream about what it would be like to travel the healing path in community. If you are meeting with a group, have your group in mind as you answer the questions. Could your group grow into the kind of apostolic band Dr. Allender describes?

Each of the four Gospels includes somewhere in its final chapters a commissioning statement from Jesus. In Matthew it is 28:16-20 and takes place in the north country of Galilee some days after the Resurrection. In Mark it is 16:15-20 and takes place just before Jesus ascends to the Father. In Luke-Acts (a two-volume work by a single author), Luke splits it between Luke 24:45-49 and Acts 1:8. John's version occurs on the evening of the Resurrection, the first time Jesus appears to his despairing friends.

Read John 20:19-23.

1. Jesus is the Sent One from the Father. When he says in verse 21 that he is sending the disciples in the same way the Father has sent him, what do you think that sending involves?

2. To empower their work, Jesus gives them the Holy Spirit. What does the Holy Spirit enable them to do?

3. To what extent do you think John means us to understand that this commission applies to us? That is, do you think this commission was just for those apostles, or does it have some relevance to us?

Although we do not have an agora comparable to that found in Greek culture, any place can become an agora. We are to create agoras not merely for the sake of evangelism, but in order to celebrate the glory of the place, to fill it with life and delight that draws others to frequent it.

Where is your agora? Wherever your passion takes you.... The agora is wherever your heart says, "Yes, I love it here," and "No, I won't let evil win. I will stand and fight the effects of the fall."

... A universe of opportunity waits for someone who can say yes to love and no to evil and longs not merely to do good, but to enter others' stories for the sake of glory.

The healing path is first and last about engagement. It is through engagement with you that I learn to hope more deeply for us. It is through hope that God slowly heals past brokenness on the basis of future promise. The healing path takes me from living as an "insider" to engaging in areas of burden and passion on the fringe of what most people view as the formal, structured local church.

—Dan Allender in THE HEALING PATH

4. When you think about going out into the agora with a band of friends, what obstacles come to mind? List as many as you can think of.

5. What are the risks involved? What would it cost you?

6. Why would anyone do this, given the obstacles, risks, and costs?

7. What help would you need?

8. The engineer in chapter 11 was afraid to ask for help from anyone. He was ashamed to need, want, desire, or dream. How does such shame hinder us from venturing out into the agora?

9. Where is your agora? Where is a place in which your heart says, "Yes, I love it here," and "No, I won't let evil win"? If you don't have such a place now, how would you go about looking?

Why did Jesus stack his apostolic band with brothers from the same family, political enemies, and wild men? After all, one of the first basic principles of the world is "avoid conflict at all costs." Join with people who are like you, hold the same core values, know the right way to dress, and accept the rules, written and unspoken. Join a club. The gospel comes along and says, "You are meant to be fools. Strangers. Pilgrims and aliens. Reenter the world and witness to my love by loving those with whom you would not normally get along." We are to join with our motley crew members and enter the agora, intending to do more than merely have a good night out and kill some time.

—Dan Allender in THE HEALING PATH

10. Understanding that God might be calling you to team up with people who are frighteningly or annoyingly different from you, take a minute to ask him to show you who those people might be. If you already have a sense of even one or two names, write them down.

Dr. Allender describes three qualities of the relationships among those who cleave together to enter the agora:

Availability and faith. "True faith remembers. Faith remembers the moments of embrace and the sweetness of reconciliation: As I have been loved, I am called to remain open to you. To open my heart to you is to be ready and willing to come to your aid with all that I have in order to do you good. It is also to open my heart to see how I have hurt you and failed to love you as well as I take care of myself. Ultimately, availability is a hunger to be forgiven, and an openness to bless and forgive."

Responsibility and hope. "Most of us are observers of life, like those who sit in the stands and watch *others* play. We feel something when we see television's images of shattered lives, but our emotions are drowned out by the next news story that passes our information-glutted eyes. To be 'response-able' is to lean into the pending redemption that is hurtling toward us at increasing speed.

"To be 'response-able' is to live with our senses alive, to gather data given to us by others and then respond to it in terms of achieving the greatest pleasure and privilege known to humankind: growing glory. Hope makes us supple and playful. Our hearts are ready and anticipating the next moment. Hope frees us to respond—to be 'response-able' to new data and new opportunities that lead to far greater joy than we normally associate with the concept of responsibility."

Accountability and love. "Accountability is storytelling in a round that brings each voice into play, ultimately forming a chorus that sings in praise of forgiveness, glories in the harvest to come, and rests in the gratitude of a day done."

11. Give an example of how you might act with each of the following in one of your relationships.

    a. availability

b. responsibility

c. accountability

12. Having reflected on the costs and value of involving yourself in a committed community, what (if anything) attracts you to the idea?

13. Are you attracted enough to pursue it? Why or why not?

Human relationships should drive us to distraction and to worship. The more involved we are with any person, the more we need God. Our joint failures and sin will lead us either to divide or to cling to God more tenaciously. The more we cling to God, the more we will turn to each other—available and broken, "response-able" and playful, accountable and at rest. The more moments of rest we enjoy with others, the more we will be in awe of them, grateful for their love.

Awe and gratitude are the fundamental building blocks of worship.

—Dan Allender in THE HEALING PATH

---

14. Spend some time thanking God for the people in
    your life who spur you on to faith, hope, and love.
    Let your gratitude move you to worship.

If you are meeting with a group, take some time for the
following activities to bring closure to your study:

- Discuss whether you want to continue
  together, perhaps with a view toward cleav-
  ing together to go out into the agora. Talk
  about what that might involve.
- Celebrate your time together. Whether you
  are going to continue or not, plan a party to
  celebrate the journey you have already made
  together. Include food and fun. Give each
  person a chance to tell what this group has
  given to him or her.
- Worship God together. You could hold
  hands and pray, sing one or more songs, or
  celebrate Communion—do whatever fits
  your customs and your situation.

32260566R00059

Made in the USA
Lexington, KY
15 May 2014